ADHD MANAGEMENT GUIDE FOR KIDS.

Your ADHD Toolbox: Essential Skills and Resources for Kids with ADHD.

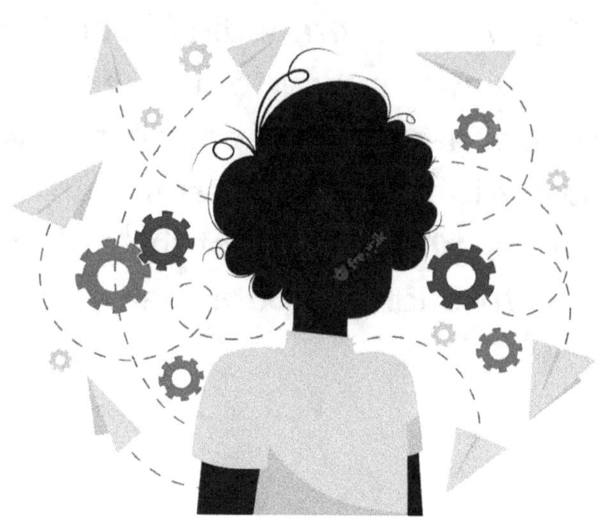

CHARLES MURRAY

TABLE OF CONTENT

INTRODUCTION.

A boy named Alex used to reside in a little village tucked away among rolling hills. Although Alex was a bright and inquisitive youngster, he frequently found it difficult to concentrate in class or complete the activities that were given to him. His parents had noted that he was easily distracted and forgetful at home, and his teachers had noted that he had trouble focusing and paying attention.

After a particularly difficult parent-teacher conference one day, Alex's parents made the decision to bring him in for an evaluation by a specialist. Alex was given the diagnosis of ADHD, a condition that affects many children and adults globally, following a number of appointments and evaluations.

Alex's parents and he initially felt relieved to finally have a reason for his troubles. They soon discovered, though, that they knew little about ADHD and how to properly manage it. To understand as much as they could about ADHD, they started reading books and articles, going to workshops and support groups, and talking to medical specialists.

They learned that there were numerous misconceptions regarding ADHD as they made their way through this unfamiliar environment and that treating the illness required a multifaceted strategy. They learnt about treatment choices for Alex's symptoms, behavioral therapy, and lifestyle modifications that could enhance his general functioning.

As Alex and his family gained experience managing ADHD, they discovered that many other families were dealing with the same difficulties they had. In an effort to help other families better understand and manage ADHD, they made the decision to create a book to share their experiences and thoughts. As a result, the "ADHD Management Guide for Kids" was created, containing helpful advice, methods, and tools to support kids and families in thriving in spite of the difficulties caused by ADHD.

CHAPTER ONE.

Understanding ADHD: What Is It and How Does It Affect Kids?.

ADHD, or Attention-Deficit/Hyperactivity Disorder, is a neurodevelopmental disorder that affects millions of children worldwide. It is characterized by symptoms of inattention, hyperactivity, and impulsivity, which can cause significant challenges in academic, social, and emotional domains.

In this chapter, we will explore what ADHD is and how it affects kids. We will discuss the symptoms of ADHD, the different types of ADHD, and the diagnostic criteria used to identify the condition. Additionally, we will explore some of the potential causes and risk factors for ADHD.

ADHD Symptoms:

The daily functioning and wellbeing of a child can be greatly impacted by ADHD symptoms. The type of ADHD a child has will determine the specific symptoms that may appear.

Attentional Problems

Children who have ADHD may struggle to focus, make careless mistakes in their homework, and have a hard time following directions. They could find it difficult to stay concentrated on work or they might be quickly distracted by outside stimuli like noise or movement. Additionally, children with ADHD may struggle to efficiently manage their time, complete assignments, and organize their things.

ADHD Signs and Symptoms
Fidgeting, restlessness, and an inability to sit still are some signs of hyperactivity. Even when it is unnecessary or inappropriate to move, children with ADHD may feel restless. They may talk too much, run or climb too much, and have trouble playing peacefully.

Irritability Signs
Children with ADHD may struggle to wait their turn, interrupt others, and answer questions before they are fully posed. They might behave rashly or without carefully considering the implications in order to satisfy their impulsive needs.

Multiple Symptoms
The most typical form of ADHD is the mixed kind, which also includes signs of impulsivity and hyperactivity. A variety of symptoms, such as forgetfulness, disorganization, fidgeting, and impulsive behaviors, may be problematic for kids with combined ADHD.

While some of these behaviors may occasionally be displayed by all kids, it's crucial to remember that signs of ADHD in kids tend to be more severe, frequent, and disruptive. Furthermore, the severity and duration of ADHD symptoms can alter over time, making proper diagnosis and continuing monitoring essential for efficient management.

Types of ADHD:

There are three forms of ADHD, or Attention-Deficit/Hyperactivity Disorder: the largely inattentive type, the mostly hyperactive-impulsive type, and the mixed type. Each variety has a distinct set of symptoms and might have a varied impact on kids.

Generally Distracted Type

Children with ADHD of the mainly inattentive kind may have trouble focusing, adhering to directions, and finishing tasks. They can find it difficult to maintain their attention on one task for an extended amount of time and are frequently diverted. They might also have trouble planning ahead and staying organized, which makes them prone to overlooking crucial information like deadlines or appointments.

Children who exhibit these symptoms of ADHD may be misdiagnosed as sluggish or unmotivated because they appear daydreamy or forgetful.

Hyperactive-Impulsive Type Is Prevalent
Children with ADHD who are predominately hyperactive-impulsive may have trouble controlling their impulsivity and inappropriate behavior. They could find it difficult to wait their turn or stay quietly, and they might always be moving. They may struggle with impulse control, speak rudely, and interrupt others. The appearance of these children with ADHD may be excessive activity or disruption, and they may be perceived as being challenging to manage or control.

Variety Type

The most prevalent kind of ADHD is the mixed form, which includes both inattentional and hyperactive-impulsive symptomatology. These symptoms may include forgetfulness, disorganization, fidgeting, impulsivity, and hyperactivity in children with this kind of ADHD. Children who have this form of ADHD may appear impulsive, restless, and quickly distracted. They may also have trouble finishing chores or paying attention to instructions.

It is crucial to remember that ADHD is a complicated disorder, and that each person will experience its symptoms differently. While some kids may only show signs of one form of ADHD, others might show signs of numerous types. Additionally, as symptoms might alter over time, a precise diagnosis and continuing observation are essential for efficient care. Understanding the many forms of ADHD can aid parents, educators, and medical professionals in identifying and meeting the special requirements of children who suffer from this illness.

Diagnosis:

Because symptoms of Attention-Deficit/Hyperactivity Disorder (ADHD) can be subtle, fluctuate in intensity, and be readily confused with typical childhood behaviors, diagnosing ADHD can be difficult. Typically, the diagnostic procedure entails a thorough evaluation that includes a medical and family history, behavioral observation, and rating scales filled out by parents, teachers, and other caregivers.

Health and Family Background

A thorough medical and family history is obtained as the first stage in the diagnosis of ADHD. This contains details about the child's growth, birth background, health issues, medication usage, and any ancestry of ADHD or other mental health issues. By identifying any hereditary or environmental factors that might be contributing to the child's symptoms, this information aids in excluding other illnesses that can resemble the symptoms of ADHD.

Observation of behavior

A crucial step in the diagnostic process is observing the child's behavior in various contexts. This could involve being observed at work, at home, or in a healthcare environment. The doctor will search for signs of impulsivity, hyperactivity, and inattention as well as any other possible behavioral or emotional problems.

Rating matrices

Parents, teachers, and other caregivers fill out questionnaires called rating scales to evaluate a child's behavior and symptoms. These scales are crucial for diagnosing ADHD since they offer details on the child's behavior in various contexts and can be used to pinpoint particular symptoms.

A thorough evaluation is necessary to make an accurate diagnosis of ADHD because there is no one-size-fits-all method for making this determination. Additional testing, such as psychological or neuropsychological evaluations, may occasionally be required to exclude alternative diagnoses or find any underlying cognitive or learning issues that might be causing the child's symptoms. After a diagnosis has been made, a treatment strategy can be created to cater to the child's particular requirements and promote their general wellbeing.

Causes and Risk Factors:

It is unclear exactly what causes Attention-Deficit/Hyperactivity Disorder (ADHD). However, research indicates that the illness might occur as a result of a mix of genetic, environmental, and neurological factors.

Genetic Variables

According to studies, ADHD tends to run in families, which raises the possibility that hereditary factors may contribute to its development. Although the precise nature of these correlations is still unclear, research has found numerous genes that may be linked to ADHD.

Environmental Elements

The emergence of ADHD may also be influenced by environmental variables. ADHD risk may be increased by exposure to pollutants like lead or alcohol during pregnancy or infancy. The likelihood of having the disease may also be increased by additional variables such low birth weight, early birth, and maternal stress during pregnancy.

psychological aspects
Additionally, studies have revealed that individuals with ADHD may have different brain structures and functions. For instance, persons with ADHD may have reduced activity in the brain regions in charge of attention, impulse control, and executive function.

Other Risk Elements
The possibility of having ADHD may also be increased by certain factors. A history of traumatic brain injury, exposure to great stress or adversity, and certain medical illnesses like sleep apnea or thyroid issues are some of these.

It is crucial to remember that ADHD is a complicated condition, and many different variables are probably responsible for its onset. Furthermore, not every person with ADHD has the same risk factors, and having one or more risk factors does not guarantee that a kid will develop ADHD. Understanding the possible causes and risk factors for ADHD can assist parents and healthcare professionals in identifying kids who may be more susceptible to the condition and in creating efficient preventative and treatment plans.

CHAPTER TWO.

Medications for ADHD: What Are the Options and How Do They Work?.

Medications are a commonly used treatment option for ADHD, or Attention-Deficit/Hyperactivity Disorder. They work by improving the function of certain neurotransmitters in the brain, which can help to reduce symptoms such as inattention, hyperactivity, and impulsivity. There are several different types of medications that are commonly used to treat ADHD, each with its own unique benefits and potential side effects.

Stimulants:

One of the most frequently recommended forms of drugs for treating ADHD, or Attention-Deficit/Hyperactivity Disorder, is stimulant medication. They function by raising dopamine and norepinephrine levels in the brain, which can enhance focus, attention, and impulse control.

Stimulants come in a variety of formulations, including short-acting and long-acting versions, and are typically thought to be safe and effective. Methylphenidate (found in products like Ritalin and Concerta) and amphetamines (found in products like Adderall and Vyvanse) are examples of stimulant drugs.

Long-acting stimulants are normally taken only once day, while short-acting stimulants are typically taken two to three times daily. Because they have fewer side effects and offer more constant symptom alleviation, long-acting versions are frequently favored. Short-acting formulations, though, may work better for some people.

Although they are typically minor and tend to go away with time as the body becomes used to the medicine, stimulant side effects are possible with some stimulant medications. Decreased appetite, difficulty sleeping, irritability, and stomach trouble are typical adverse effects. Rarely, stimulant drugs might result in more severe adverse effects like accelerated heart rate, hypertension, or symptoms of psychosis.

Children who are taking stimulant drugs for ADHD need to be constantly monitored by their parents and medical professionals, and any concerns about side effects or changes in symptoms need to be shared. Additionally, because stimulant drugs might occasionally influence these characteristics, it is important to keep an eye on the growth and weight gain of children who are taking them.

Although many children with ADHD can benefit greatly from stimulant drugs, they are not suitable for everyone. It may not be possible for children to use stimulant drugs if they have specific medical disorders, such as heart issues or uncontrolled high blood pressure. Additionally, some kids could react poorly to stimulant drugs or might have serious adverse effects. Non-stimulant drugs or other therapy approaches may be thought of in such circumstances.

Non-Stimulant Medications:

For those with ADHD who do not respond favorably to or are unable to handle stimulant drugs, non-stimulant meds offer an alternate therapy option. These drugs function by raising norepinephrine levels in the brain, which can enhance focus and restrain impulses.

Atomoxetine (Strattera) and guanfacine (Intuniv) are two non-stimulant drugs for ADHD that are frequently prescribed. Guanfacine is only permitted for use in children and adolescents, whereas atomoxetine is permitted for use in both children and adults.

The effects of atomoxetine, which is normally taken once daily, may not be felt for several weeks. It has been demonstrated to be useful in reducing signs of inattention and hyperactivity, albeit for some people, it might not be as effective as stimulant drugs. Stomach upset, decreased appetite, and weariness are typical atomoxetine adverse effects.

Guanfacine is normally taken once day and is frequently used in conjunction with stimulant drugs as a complementary therapy. It has been proven to be successful in reducing impulsivity and hyperactive symptoms, and it might also help with sleep problems and anxiety symptoms. Guanfacine frequently causes stomach discomfort, dizziness, and sleepiness as adverse effects.

For people who take stimulant medications frequently and experience serious adverse effects or who have certain medical problems that make stimulant medications dangerous, non-stimulant medications can be a better choice. They might also be favored in cases when co-occurring disorders like anxiety or tic disorders are present because stimulant medicines may make them worse.

It's crucial to remember that non-stimulant drugs might not work as well for everyone with ADHD and might take longer to start showing results than stimulant meds. In order to guarantee that a medicine is working as intended and that any side effects are properly treated, close monitoring and communication with healthcare professionals are essential.

Other Medications:

There are other drugs that may be used to treat ADHD in some people in addition to stimulant and non-stimulant drugs. These medicines consist of:

Alpha-2 agonists: These drugs, such as guanfacine (Intuniv) and clonidine, are normally used to treat high blood pressure, but they can also be useful in lowering symptoms of hyperactivity, impulsivity, and aggression in people with ADHD.

Antidepressants: People who also have anxiety or depression may benefit from taking some antidepressants, such as bupropion and tricyclic antidepressants, to manage their ADHD. Additionally, these drugs might aid with impulse and attention control.

Antipsychotics: In some situations, people with severe hyperactivity or aggressive symptoms associated with ADHD may be treated with antipsychotic drugs. These drugs, meanwhile, can have serious negative effects and are normally only prescribed to people who don't react to conventional forms of treatment.

These drugs are not regarded first-line therapies for ADHD and are typically only prescribed to people who do not respond well to or are unable to take stimulant or non-stimulant drugs. To enhance general symptom management, they may also be used in conjunction with other therapies, such as behavioral therapy.

As with other medications, it is crucial to constantly monitor people who are taking them for ADHD, and to let medical professionals know if there are any concerns or changes in symptoms. People should also be aware of any possible adverse effects linked with these medications and should talk to their healthcare provider if they have any concerns.

CHAPTER THREE.

Behavioral Therapy for ADHD: How Can It Help Kids Manage Symptoms?.

A form of therapy that can be used to help people with ADHD control their symptoms is behavioral therapy, which is often referred to as behavior modification or behavior management. This kind of therapy focuses on altering particular troublesome behaviors and can support people in learning new abilities and symptom-management techniques.

Working with a therapist or counselor who specializes in treating ADHD with behavioral therapy is normal. The therapist will collaborate with the patient and their family to identify specific troublesome behaviors, such as impulsivity or trouble paying attention, and will create a strategy for dealing with these behaviors.

Following are a few typical techniques used in behavioral therapy for ADHD:

Positive reinforcement:

Positive reinforcement is a method for changing behavior that involves rewarding desired actions to make them more likely to be repeated in the future. This strategy is based on the idea that rewarding activities are more likely to be repeated, but unrewarding behaviors are less likely to be repeated.

Positive reinforcement can be a particularly successful strategy for promoting desired behaviors in the setting of ADHD, such as paying attention in class, finishing homework on time, or following instructions. In this situation, positive reinforcement approaches like the following could be applied:

Verbal acclaim: This entails verbally thanking the person for displaying desired behaviour. A teacher might commend a pupil for raising their hand and waiting their turn to speak in class, for instance.

For displaying desired actions, tangible rewards can be given in the form of a sticker or tiny toy. For instance, a parent might offer a little incentive for submitting homework on time.

Granting exceptional privileges, such additional screen time or the option to select a preferred activity, as a reward for displaying desired behaviors falls under this category of privileges.

For people with ADHD, positive reinforcement can be an effective approach since it can encourage them to display desired behaviors and boost their self-esteem and confidence. It's crucial to regularly utilize positive reinforcement and to cater the incentives to the needs and interests of the individual. Negative repercussions or punishment should also be avoided because they might be demotivating and create unfavorable linkages between desired activities.

Token economies:

A sort of behavior modification strategy known as token economics includes rewarding good conduct with tokens, points, or other benefits. This method is frequently employed in therapeutic and educational contexts to motivate people with ADHD to display desired behaviors, such as paying attention in class or finishing their schoolwork on time.

In a token economy, the person receives rewards for engaging in desired activities in the form of tokens or points. Then, these tokens can be traded in for benefits like more screen time, a favorite snack, or other privileges. The incentives are often something that the person finds motivating and pleasurable and are chosen based on their interests and needs.

One advantage of a token economy is that it may be a very powerful tool for promoting beneficial behaviors, especially when used repeatedly over time. For people with ADHD, token economies can be especially helpful since they offer fast, clear feedback on behavior and can boost motivation and self-esteem.

However, in order for a token economy to work well, it must be used properly. Key pointers for utilizing a token economy are as follows:

Select the right incentives: Incentives should be motivating and enjoyable to the recipient and should be suited to his or her interests and needs.

Be consistent: In order to reinforce desirable behavior, rewards should be given frequently and right away after the behavior.

Use a clear system: The token economy's rules should be simple to grasp and the individual should be aware of the actions that will earn rewards.

Fade the tokens: As the person starts to regularly display the required behaviors without the need for rewards, the use of tokens should be gradually phased out over time.

In general, a token economy can be an effective tool for ADHD sufferers, especially when combined with other behavior modification methods and tactics. A token economy can boost motivation and self-esteem by giving clear feedback and rewarding good conduct. It can also motivate people with ADHD to learn new skills and techniques for controlling their symptoms.

Time management and organizational skills:

For people with ADHD, time management and organizational skills are crucial because issues with these abilities can frequently result in issues with finishing projects, meeting deadlines, and managing daily duties. To better control their symptoms and excel in school, the workplace, and daily life, people with

ADHD can learn to acquire efficient time management and organizational skills with the correct tools and assistance.

Some techniques for helping people with ADHD gain time-management and organization skills include:

Making use of a planner or calendar: People with ADHD can benefit from using a planner or calendar to remember due dates, appointments, and other significant occasions. Whether using a paper planner, a digital calendar, or a hybrid of the two, it is crucial to pick a system that works well for the individual.

Tasks should be broken down into smaller pieces because they can be daunting for people with ADHD and cause them to put off or avoid doing them. Tasks can be made more manageable and people can stay on track by breaking them up into smaller parts.

Prioritizing tasks: It's crucial for people with ADHD to order tasks according to importance and completion date. By delegating or deferring less important work, this might assist ensure that important tasks are completed on schedule.

Using reminders and alarms: People with ADHD who have forgetfulness may find benefit from using reminders and alarms. For crucial chores and appointments, setting reminders helps guarantee that they are not forgotten.

Establishing a dedicated workstation can aid people with ADHD in maintaining their attention and staying on target. It is crucial to pick a workspace that is conducive to efficiency, distraction-free, and comfortable.

Support: People with ADHD may benefit from getting guidance from a coach, counselor, or therapist who may guide them in building strong organizational and time management skills.

In general, improving organizational and time management skills is a crucial part of treating ADHD symptoms. People with ADHD can learn to better control their symptoms and accomplish their goals by employing techniques including using a planner or calendar, breaking things down into smaller pieces, and prioritizing chores.

Parent training:

An evidence-based strategy known as parent training assists parents of children with ADHD in creating efficient symptom management and daily functioning plans for their children. In most parent education programs, parents attend a number of sessions where they learn about ADHD, its signs and symptoms, and how it affects their child's behavior and development. Additionally, they pick up useful techniques like time-outs, positive reinforcement, and effective communication for controlling their child's behavior.

Numerous delivery methods, such as group sessions, one-on-one coaching, and online courses, are available for parent education programs. Peer support is another feature of certain systems, allowing parents to network with other parents facing comparable difficulties.

Focusing on creating strong bonds between parents and their kids is one of the fundamental tenets of parent education. This includes avoiding negative actions like criticism or punishment and employing positive reinforcement to promote good conduct. The need of consistency in parenting and creating clear, consistent standards and expectations for behavior are other points that are emphasized in parent training.

The behavior and functioning of kids with ADHD can be improved, according to studies, with parent instruction. Children who receive therapy through parent training demonstrate improvements in their ADHD symptoms, social skills, and academic achievement. Parents who participate in parent training programs report feeling more secure in their abilities to manage their child's behavior.

In general, parent training is a crucial part of ADHD treatment and can be a helpful tool for parents who are having trouble controlling their child's symptoms. Parent training can assist to improve the quality of life for both parents and children by giving them the knowledge and abilities they need to effectively manage their child's behavior.

CHAPTER FOUR.

Nutrition and ADHD: How Does Diet Affect Symptoms?.

Nutrition plays an important role in overall health and wellbeing, and research has shown that it can also affect symptoms of ADHD. While diet alone is not a substitute for medical treatment, making certain dietary changes can help to manage symptoms and improve overall health.

One factor that may contribute to ADHD symptoms is blood sugar levels. Eating foods high in sugar or carbohydrates can cause blood sugar levels to spike, followed by a crash in energy and concentration.

To help manage blood sugar levels and reduce ADHD symptoms, it is recommended to eat a balanced diet that includes complex carbohydrates, healthy fats, and protein.

Some foods that may be particularly beneficial for individuals with ADHD include:

Protein-rich foods:

A critical component of numerous body processes, including tissue growth and repair, the synthesis of hormones and enzymes, and immune system maintenance, protein is a necessary macronutrient. Getting adequate protein in your diet is crucial for ADHD sufferers since it can aid with focus, attention, and mood.

There are numerous protein-rich foods available, both from animal and plant sources. Meats like beef, chicken, and pork are examples of animal-based sources of protein, along with fish and eggs. In addition to being strong in protein, these meals also provide vital elements including iron, zinc, and vitamin B12.

Among the protein-rich plant foods include nuts, seeds, beans, and lentils. In addition to being strong in protein, these foods are also high in fiber and other vital nutrients. Tofu and tempeh are examples of soy products that are excellent providers of plant-based protein.

Lean sources of protein, such as skinless chicken breast or lean beef cuts, should be used to provide protein to meals. Overconsumption of saturated fat and cholesterol, which can harm the heart, can be avoided in this way.

The general quality of the protein in the diet must also be taken into account. For instance, plant-based proteins might not include all the essential amino acids required for optimum health, making them incomplete. However, people can make a complete protein diet by combining several plant-based proteins, such as rice and beans or peanut butter and whole grain bread.

In conclusion, including protein-rich foods in the diet can assist to manage ADHD symptoms and improve general health. People can make sure they are obtaining the nutrients they need for optimal health by selecting lean sources of protein and including a variety of animal and plant-based sources.

Complex carbohydrates:

For those with ADHD, complex carbs are an essential nutrient. These kinds of carbs provide a consistent and sustained source of energy throughout the day since they digest more gradually than simple carbohydrates. This can lessen energy and mood dips that might otherwise have a detrimental effect on concentration and focus.

Various foods, including whole grains, vegetables, and fruits, contain complex carbs. Complex carbs can be found in abundance in whole grains like brown rice, quinoa, and whole grain bread. Additionally, the high fiber content of these foods can aid in better digestion and blood sugar control.

Sweet potatoes, squash, and carrots are a few examples of vegetables that are excellent suppliers of complex carbs. Not only are these foods nutrient-dense, but they also offer significant fiber and antioxidants.

A fantastic source of complex carbohydrates include fruits like berries, apples, and bananas. Additionally, these foods include significant amounts of vitamins and minerals, which are essential for good health and wellbeing.

The distinction between different types of carbohydrates must be made. Simple carbs, such as those found in processed foods and sugary beverages, can increase blood sugar levels, which can exacerbate ADHD symptoms. Therefore, wherever possible, it's crucial to prefer complex carbohydrates over simple ones.

In conclusion, adding complex carbs to the diet can assist to reduce ADHD symptoms and improve general health. People can make sure they are obtaining the nutrients they need to thrive by choosing whole grains, veggies, and fruits.

Omega-3 fatty acids:

Polyunsaturated fatty acids, such as omega-3 fatty acids, are crucial for overall health and well-being. These fats are essential for the growth and upkeep of the neurological system, which is important for brain function. Omega-3 fatty acids can enhance general brain health in people with ADHD by enhancing cognitive function, reducing inflammation, and supporting cognitive function.

Alpha-linolenic acid (ALA), eicosapentaenoic acid (EPA), and docosahexaenoic acid (DHA) are the three different kinds of omega-3 fatty acids. While EPA and DHA are mostly found in cold-water fish like salmon, mackerel, and sardines, ALA is found in plant-based sources including flaxseeds, chia seeds, and walnuts.

According to research, EPA and DHA, two omega-3 fatty acids, can aid both children and adults with ADHD by reducing their symptoms. According to studies, taking supplements of these fatty acids can aid with concentration, focus, and general cognitive function.

Omega-3 fatty acids contain anti-inflammatory qualities that can aid in reducing inflammation throughout the body in addition to improving brain function. ADHD is one of many health issues that have been connected to chronic inflammation. Omega-3 fatty acids can enhance general health and well-being by lowering inflammation.

Consuming meals high in these nutrients or taking supplements are two ways to add omega-3 fatty acids to your diet. For those who decide to take supplements, it's crucial to pick one with both EPA and DHA that is of a good caliber. It is advised to include plant-based sources of ALA in the diet along with eating fatty fish at least twice a week for individuals who want to get their omega-3 fatty acids from food.

In conclusion, omega-3 fatty acids are a necessary component for good health and are particularly beneficial for those with ADHD. People can aid to enhance cognitive function, lower inflammation, and support general brain health by include these healthy fats in their diets through food or supplements.

CHAPTER FIVE.

Exercise and ADHD: How Can Physical Activity Help Kids with ADHD?.

Beyond simply enhancing cognitive performance and easing symptoms, exercise has several positive effects on those with ADHD. For instance, consistent exercise can aid with sleep quality, which is frequently disturbed in people with ADHD. Exercise can help people with ADHD feel more refreshed and aware during the day by encouraging better sleep.

Additionally, exercise can aid ADHD sufferers with their social skills and self-esteem. For those with ADHD, taking part in team sports or group fitness courses might present possibilities for social interaction and social skill development. By setting and accomplishing fitness goals, exercise can also help people with ADHD feel a feeling of success and improve their self-esteem.

It's important to remember that exercise doesn't have to be difficult or have a big impact to be beneficial. For people with ADHD, even low-intensity exercise, like strolling or light stretching, might be beneficial. In fact, some studies have found that mindfulness- and relaxation-focused exercises like yoga or tai chi can be very beneficial for easing ADHD symptoms.

Finding fun and enduring activities is crucial when adding exercise into a regular schedule. This may improve commitment to and motivation for an exercise regimen. When selecting a fitness regimen, it's necessary to take into account elements like time limits, accessibility, and personal preferences.

Last but not least, it's critical to remember that exercise should not be utilized in place of other ADHD therapies like medication or behavioral therapy. But when combined with other therapies, exercise can be a potent strategy for controlling ADHD symptoms and enhancing general wellbeing.

In conclusion, regular exercise can help people with ADHD in a variety of ways, such as by enhancing cognitive function, lowering symptoms, improved sleep quality, enhancing social skills and self-esteem, and promoting both physical and mental health. People with ADHD can take charge of their health and wellbeing by finding fun and sustainable activities to engage in on a daily basis and by including exercise into their routine.

CHAPTER SIX

School and ADHD: What Are Some Classroom Accommodations and Strategies?.

Children with ADHD could have trouble focusing on work, remaining organized, and sitting still for extended periods of time in a classroom setting. Fortunately, there are lots of classroom modifications and approaches that can support these kids' intellectual and social development.

A 504 plan, a legal document that specifies the particular accommodations and assistance a child needs to succeed in school, is a popular concession for kids with ADHD. Common modifications for kids with ADHD include extra time for tests, preferred sitting close to the teacher, and lots of breaks to let off steam.

Using a visual timetable or planner to assist kids with ADHD stay organized and manage their time is another successful method of treatment. This can be done by making a daily schedule that specifies times for various activities or by utilizing a planner to keep track of tasks and due dates. Visual schedules and planners can support youngsters with ADHD in staying focused and on-task by establishing structure and routine.

There are numerous classroom-based interventions that

can assist children with ADHD achieve academically in addition to accommodations and tactics. For instance, to aid children with ADHD in understanding and memory, teachers can employ multi-sensory teaching methods such including hands-on activities or visual aids. In order to encourage and motivate students with ADHD, teachers should also offer regular positive reinforcement and incentives for good behavior, such as verbal compliments or modest gifts.

Fostering a good and supportive school atmosphere is crucial for supporting students with ADHD in the classroom. This may entail supporting neurodiversity acceptance and understanding, offering opportunity for mobility and sensory breaks, and fostering open dialogue between educators, parents, and kids.

Overall, there are lots of efficient interventions, adjustments, and tactics that can help kids with ADHD succeed in school. Children with ADHD can get the help and resources they need to succeed academically and socially by collaborating with teachers, parents, and other experts.

CHAPTER SEVEN.

Technology and ADHD: What Are Some Pros and Cons, and How Can It Be Used Wisely?.

The extensive availability and use of technology in recent years has had a profound impact on how children learn and engage with their environment. These adjustments can be both a difficulty and an opportunity for kids with ADHD.

The availability of educational applications and programs for kids with ADHD is one of the main advantages of technology. These resources can be utilized to strengthen education and raise academic performance. For instance, educational games and programs can make learning enjoyable and interesting, which can help youngsters with ADHD stay focused. Technology can also offer tools like speech-to-text software, which can aid kids who have trouble expressing themselves in writing.

Technology may also be able to assist kids with ADHD in maintaining their organization and time management. Many kids with ADHD have trouble remembering tasks, assignments, and due dates. Calendars, to-do lists, and other tools made available by technology can help people keep organized and relieve stress.

For kids with ADHD, however, digital use may also have drawbacks.

Screen time can cause overstimulation and distraction, which can make ADHD symptoms worse. Additionally, overusing social media and other online platforms can lead to anxiety and social comparison, both of which have a detrimental effect on mental health.

Setting clear guidelines and limitations for screen time is essential for technology use. The amount of time spent using devices, as well as the times and locations where they may be utilized, can all be restricted by parents and other adults. Additionally, it's critical to keep an eye on the kinds of information kids are consuming and make sure it's both age- and distraction-appropriate.

It's crucial to encourage kids with ADHD to participate in various activities that increase physical activity and social connection in addition to setting boundaries. This can include sports, pastimes, and outdoor pursuits that offer chances for exercise, interaction with others, and stress release.

Technology can be used by parents and other caregivers to support behavior management techniques including reward schemes and behavior tracking. For instance, there are apps available that let parents create digital token economies to recognize good behavior in their children.

It is crucial to remember that technology shouldn't be used in place of other therapies like medication or behavioral therapy. Instead, technology can be utilized to support these interventions as an additional tool.

In the end, the secret to helping kids with ADHD use technology effectively is to approach it with a deliberate and thinking perspective. Children with ADHD can benefit from technology while limiting any possible drawbacks by establishing clear boundaries and encouraging a healthy mix of screen time and other activities.

CHAPTER EIGHT.

Frequently Asked Questions and Answers.

What is ADHD?

ADHD stands for attention-deficit/hyperactivity disorder. It is a neurodevelopmental disorder that affects both children and adults.

What are the symptoms of ADHD?

Symptoms of ADHD include inattention, hyperactivity, and impulsivity.

How is ADHD diagnosed?

ADHD is diagnosed through a combination of evaluations, including a medical exam, parent and teacher reports, and behavioral assessments.

Can ADHD be cured?

There is no cure for ADHD, but there are effective treatments that can help manage symptoms.

What are the different types of ADHD?

There are three types of ADHD: predominantly inattentive type, predominantly hyperactive-impulsive type, and combined type.

What causes ADHD?

The exact cause of ADHD is unknown, but it is believed to be caused by a combination of genetic and environmental factors.

Is ADHD hereditary?

There is a strong genetic component to ADHD, meaning it can be inherited.

Can ADHD be treated without medication?

Yes, there are several non-medication treatments available for ADHD, including behavioral therapy, parent training, and dietary changes.

What medications are used to treat ADHD?

Stimulants and non-stimulants are the two main types of medications used to treat ADHD.

What are the side effects of ADHD medication?

Side effects of ADHD medication can include loss of appetite, insomnia, and irritability.

Can ADHD medication be addictive?

When used as prescribed, ADHD medication is not addictive. However, it can be abused if misused or taken in larger doses than prescribed.

Can children with ADHD outgrow it?

While symptoms of ADHD may improve with age, it is a lifelong condition that typically requires ongoing management.

Can children with ADHD excel academically?

Yes, with proper treatment and accommodations, children with ADHD can excel academically.

What are some accommodations that can be made for children with ADHD in the classroom?

Accommodations for children with ADHD may include preferential seating, additional time for assignments and tests, and a designated quiet space for focus.

How can parents help their child with ADHD at home?

Parents can help their child with ADHD at home by creating structure, setting clear expectations, and providing positive reinforcement for good behavior.

Can diet affect ADHD symptoms?

There is some evidence that certain dietary changes, such as increasing intake of omega-3 fatty acids, can improve ADHD symptoms.

Are there any alternative treatments for ADHD?
Some alternative treatments, such as neurofeedback and meditation, have shown promise in reducing symptoms of ADHD.

How can exercise help children with ADHD?
Exercise can help children with ADHD by providing an outlet for excess energy and improving focus and concentration.

Can children with ADHD have successful social lives?
Yes, with proper support and social skills training, children with ADHD can have successful social lives.

Can ADHD be misdiagnosed?

Yes, ADHD can be misdiagnosed, particularly if symptoms are caused by another underlying condition.

Can adults be diagnosed with ADHD?

Yes, adults can be diagnosed with ADHD, even if they were not diagnosed as children.

Can ADHD lead to other mental health issues?

Untreated ADHD can increase the risk of other mental health issues, such as anxiety and depression.

Is ADHD more common in boys or girls?

ADHD is more commonly diagnosed in boys than girls, but it is believed that the condition is equally common among both sexes.

Can adults be diagnosed with ADHD?

Yes, adults can be diagnosed with ADHD. In fact, many people with ADHD are not diagnosed until adulthood. The symptoms of ADHD can persist into adulthood and can affect many areas of life, including work, relationships, and overall quality of life.

Can ADHD be cured?

There is no cure for ADHD, but it can be managed with the right treatment and support. With proper management, many people with ADHD are able to live fulfilling and successful lives.

How do I talk to my child about their ADHD?

It is important to talk to your child about their ADHD in a way that is positive and empowering. Focus on their strengths and how they can use them to overcome challenges. You can also help them understand that ADHD is a part of who they are and does not define them as a person.

Can diet alone manage ADHD symptoms?

Diet alone is unlikely to completely manage ADHD symptoms, but it can play a role in symptom management. A healthy, balanced diet can help support overall brain function and may help improve focus and concentration. However, it is important to work with a healthcare professional to develop a comprehensive treatment plan.

Can ADHD be overdiagnosed?

There is some debate about whether ADHD is overdiagnosed, but it is important to remember that each person with ADHD is unique and deserves individualized treatment and support. Proper diagnosis and treatment can help ensure that individuals with ADHD receive the support they need to thrive.

Can ADHD medication be addictive?

ADHD medication is not addictive when used as directed and under the supervision of a healthcare professional. However, it is important to follow the prescribed dosage and not misuse or share medication.

Can ADHD be caused by bad parenting?

No, ADHD is not caused by bad parenting. ADHD is a neurodevelopmental disorder that is believed to be caused by a combination of genetic and environmental factors.

Can ADHD be managed without medication?

While medication is often a key part of ADHD treatment, there are other strategies that can be effective in managing symptoms. These may include behavioral therapy, dietary changes, exercise, and accommodations at school or work.

Can ADHD go away on its own?

ADHD is a chronic condition that does not go away on its own. However, with proper management and support, many people with ADHD are able to live successful and fulfilling lives.

Can ADHD be misdiagnosed as something else?

Yes, ADHD can sometimes be misdiagnosed as other conditions, such as anxiety, depression, or learning disabilities. This is why it is important to work with a healthcare professional who has experience diagnosing and treating ADHD. A comprehensive evaluation can help ensure an accurate diagnosis and the most effective treatment plan.

9 798393 874339